MINDFULNESS MEDITATION & YOGA

BY GRACE KIMANI

Mind, Body, Spirit- Less Stress & more peace

Table of Contents

1. Note from the Author

<u>Section one:</u>

2. Introduction to Yoga
3. The Sutra – A philosophical Guide to yoga
4. What do I need to practice yoga?
5. Why should you try yoga?
6. What are the Physical benefits of practicing yoga?
7. Basic Yoga Class:
-   Mountain Pose (Tadasana)
-   Chair Pose (Utkatasana)
-   Child Pose (Balasana)
-   Cat Pose (Marjariasana)
-   Cobra Pose (Bhujangasana)
-   Downward Facing Dog Pose (Adho Mukha Svanansana)
-   Warrior I (Virabhadrasana I)
-   Warrior II (Virabhadrasana II)
-   Seated Twist (Ardha matsyendrasana)
-   Bridge Pose (Setu Bhanda)
-   Corpse Pose (Shavasana)

<u>Section two:</u>

1. Introduction to Mindfulness
2. What are the core benefits of Mindfulness?
3. How can we practice Mindfulness?
4. Mindfulness for women and pregnancy
5. Reasons to practice mindfulness during pregnancy
6. Mindful Parenting
7. How can we rehearse to accomplish Mindful Parenting?
8. Key advantages of Mindful Parenting
9. Mindfulness for children
10. Meditation
11. Summary

Note from the Author

This book is designed to be fairly short, quick and easy to read. I like to just get to the point instead of beating round the bush. You can use these simple practices at home, incorporate them into your daily life to help with anxiety, stress, tiredness and unhappiness.

Peace can't be achieved in the outside world, unless we have peace on the inside. So let us begin our journey of finding peace within ourselves.

YOGA

Section 1 - Introduction to Yoga

What is Yoga?

Yoga is the unification of our mind and body as one. It involves three main elements. This type of yoga is called Hatha yoga.

- Breathing – Breathing control is achieved through breathing techniques known as Pranayama.
- Meditation – Meditation is used to reach a peaceful state of mind and body.
- Physical and mental exercise – Exercise is performed through physical postures or poses known as Asana.

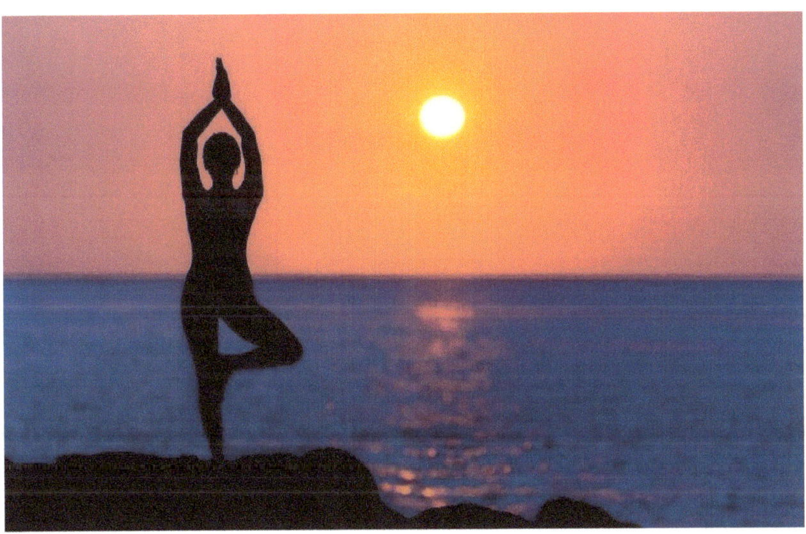

Yoga exercises improve the body's circulation and lead to the body becoming healthier and more efficient.

Through breath control, you can increase mind and body functionality. Yoga exercises combined with breathing controlled skills prepare the mind and body for meditation. In turn, meditation helps the mind and body to be free from stress and anxiety. Regularly practiced, the three elements of yoga help bring about the clarity of mind and a strong, capable body.

The Sutra – A philosophical Guide to yoga

The Sutra is a collection of 196 principles, acting as a philosophical guide for a yogi. The Sutra outlines the eight limbs of yoga.

1. Yama – rules of morality
2. Niyama – Observances / habitual activities for healthy living
3. Asanas – Physical postures or poses
4. Pranayama – Controlled breathing
5. Pratyahara – Controlling sight, sound, smell, taste, and touch, to reach enlightenment
6. Dharana – Concentration or single focus
7. Dhyana – meditation
8. Samadhi – state of intense concentration, absorption

What do I need to practice yoga?

- Your body, an open mind and a sense of intrigue.
- Wear something comfortable that you can move freely in, and you don't need any shoes as yoga is practiced barefoot.
- A yoga mat
- Don't practice on a full stomach as there are lots of bending and twisting of the body.

Why should you try yoga?

- Help you with a better sleep routine
- It can prevent you from catching a cold
- Give you a sense of ease and calm
- Improve your health
- Help heal aches and pains

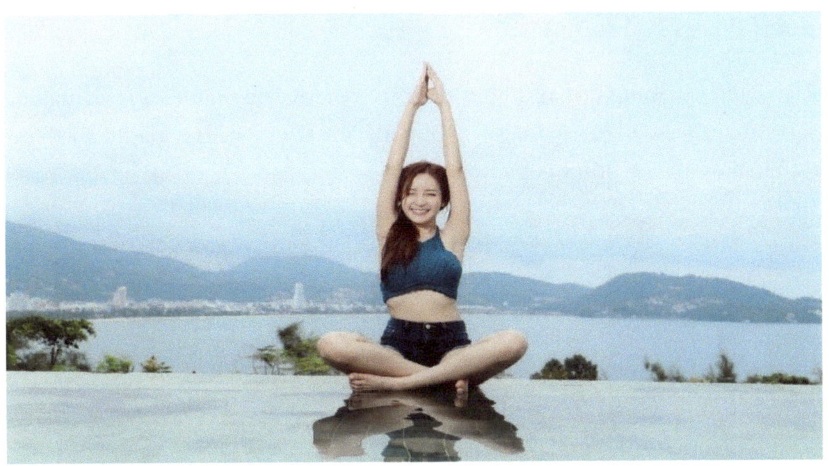

What are the Physical benefits of practicing yoga?

- Improvement in your flexibility after a few weeks of practicing yoga. This will also improve your posture, as your muscles and ligaments are less tight. Tight muscles can add strain to areas such as knees, thighs, shinbone, and spine.
- You will see a great improvement in your muscle strength which is a great benefit as you will have protection from conditions such as arthritis and severe back pain.
- Bad posture is responsible for many problems relating to the neck, back, shoulders and knee joints. Yoga will help you improve your posture and give you the correct support. Postures performed through yoga exercises can help strengthen bone, increase density and help retain calcium.
- Yoga prevents joint and cartilage wear and tear which is a great benefit. By doing certain yoga exercises which give the joint areas a thorough workout. Working the joint areas through their full motion range will make sure the cartilage is fully nourished.
- Increased circulation will improve as physical exercises performed during yoga will help oxygenate and thin our blood cells. All areas of the body will receive freshly oxygenated blood through the different movements.

Basic Yoga Class:

Here I have compiled some very friendly Yoga positions that will help you ease into the splendid art of Yoga.

Mountain Pose (Tadasana)

'Tada' means a mountain and that's from where the name is originated. Tadasana mainly involves a major group of muscles and is marked as the starting pose of all the other yoga positions.

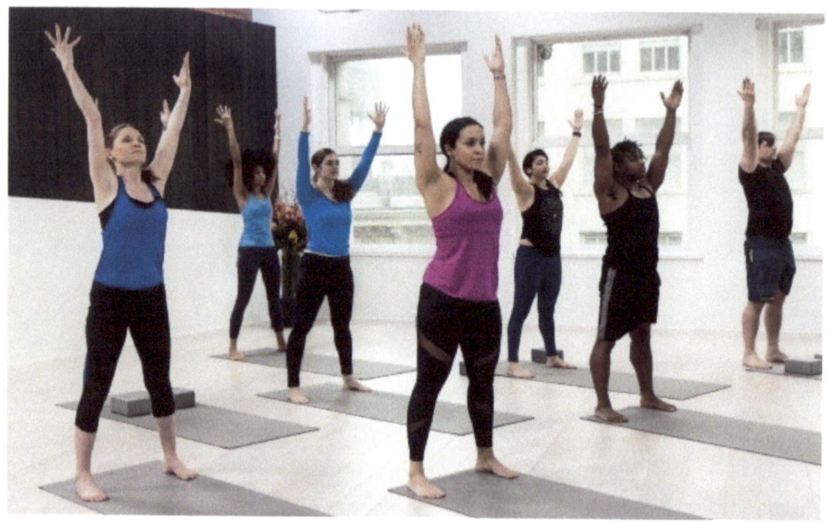

- **Benefits of Mountain Pose:**
  - ➤ Improves posture
  - ➤ Progresses focus and concentration
  - ➤ Sense of centre
  - ➤ Mental clarity
  - ➤ Solid breathing exercise
- **How to do it?**
  - ➤ Stand with your feet tall and arms at your side
  - ➤ Ground your feet in such a way that all four corners press into the ground.
  - ➤ Balance your body weight on your feet.
  - ➤ Then take a deep breath and raise your hands overhead
  - ➤ Palms should be facing each other with arms straight.
  - ➤ Now Exhale you release arms back to your sides

Chair Pose (Utkatasana):

Chair pose strengthens the muscles of your legs and arms. It can boost your energy levels and enhances your willpower.

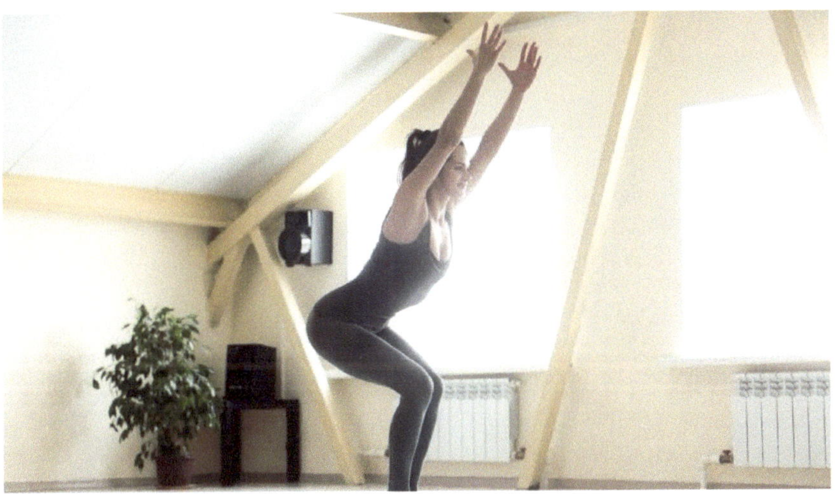

- **Benefits of Chair Pose:**
  - Tones up your leg muscles brilliantly
  - Toughens hip flexors, ankles, calves, and back
  - Stretches chest and shoulders
  - Reduces symptoms of flat feet
- **How to do it?**
  - Stand straight with your feet apart.
  - Stretch your hands to the front with your palms facing downwards. Remember, your elbows should not bend
  - Bend your knees.
  - Gently push your pelvis down as if you are sitting in an imaginary chair.
  - Hold the pose and take deep breaths.
  - To end up the pose, straighten your legs on an inhale, and bring your arms to your sides in an exhale

Child Pose (Balasana):

Child Pose is one of the easiest poses that relaxes your nervous system and calms you down. For its best practice, just close your eyes and listen to your breath.

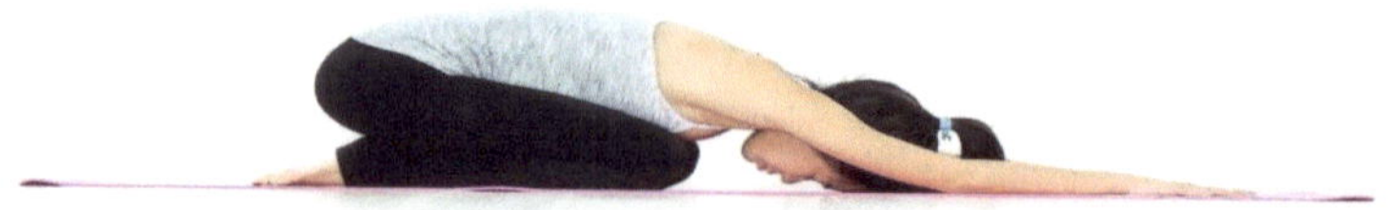

- **Benefits of Child Pose:**
  - Stretches hips, thighs, and ankles.
  - Relieves back and neck pain.
  - Restores your energies physically, mentally and emotionally
  - Let you relax.
- **How to do it?**
  - Firstly, you need to bend your knees and sit on your heels.
  - Your hips should be firmly placed on your heels.
  - Next, lower your head on to the mat and bring your hands forward by your side.
  - Press your thighs against your chest and breathe lightly.

Cat Pose (Marjariasana):

Cat pose promotes spinal flexibility and provides a perfect massage to your belly organs. It is valuable both for the beginners as well as the advanced experts.

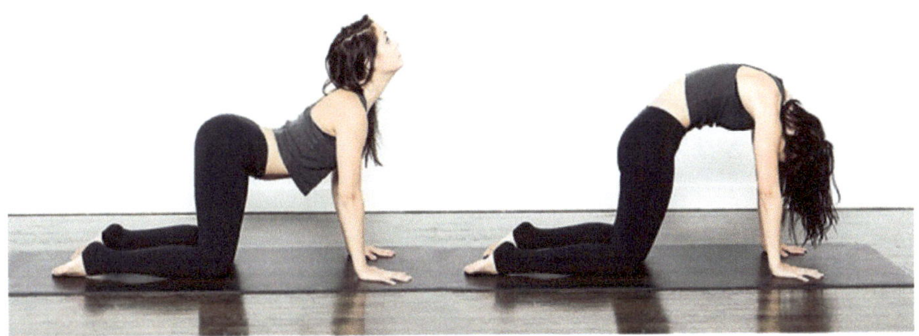

- **Benefits of Cat Pose:**
- ➢ Improved emotional balance
- ➢ Stability of the mind
- ➢ Tones up the gastrointestinal tract
- ➢ Increases the adaptability of neck, shoulders, and spine
- ➢ Lowers back pain
- **How to do it?**
- ➢ Stand on all fours, such that your back forms a table top and your feet and hands from its legs.
- ➢ Your arms should be perpendicular to the floor.
- ➢ Place your hands flat on the floor right under the shoulders.
- ➢ Your knees should be placed hip-width apart.
- ➢ Look straight ahead.
- ➢ Inhale and raise your chin as you tilt your head backward. Push your navel down and raise your tailbone. Compress your buttocks. You might feel a tingling sensation.
- ➢ Hold the pose for a few breaths. Breathe long and deep.
- ➢ Next, exhale and drop your chin to your chest as you arch your back and relax your buttocks.
- ➢ Hold this position for a few breaths. Then, back to the tabletop position.

Cobra Pose (Bhujangasana):

Are you stressed out? Are you sick of your stiff back and also that baggy belly? Practicing cobra pose is perfect at this point.

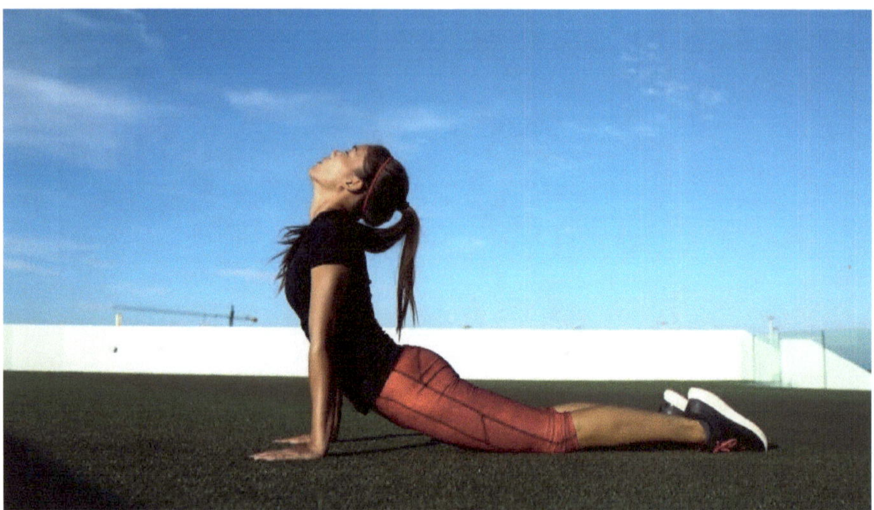

- **Benefits of Cobra Pose:**
- ➢ Good for kidney
- ➢ Prevent thyroid problems
- ➢ Treats back pain
- ➢ Enhance digestion process
- ➢ Good for asthma patients.
- ➢ Reduce belly fats
- ➢ Manages stress
- ➢ Elevates moods
- ➢ Beneficial for the slipped disc patients.
- **How to do it?**
- ➢ Lay face-down on the floor and extend your legs behind you, spread a few inches apart.
- ➢ Place your hands in a way that your fingers are pointing toward the top of the mat.
- ➢ Put your elbows on the sides of your body.
- ➢ Inhale as you gently lift your head and chest off the floor. Keep your lower ribs on the floor.
- ➢ Gaze at the sky.
- ➢ Hold the pose for about 30 seconds.

➢ To release from this position, exhale and slowly lower your chest and forehead to the mat.

Downward Facing Dog Pose (Adho Mukha Svanansana):

Downward facing dog pose is a perfect way to stretch your back, arms, shoulders; almost everything. It gets you centered, calm and peaceful.

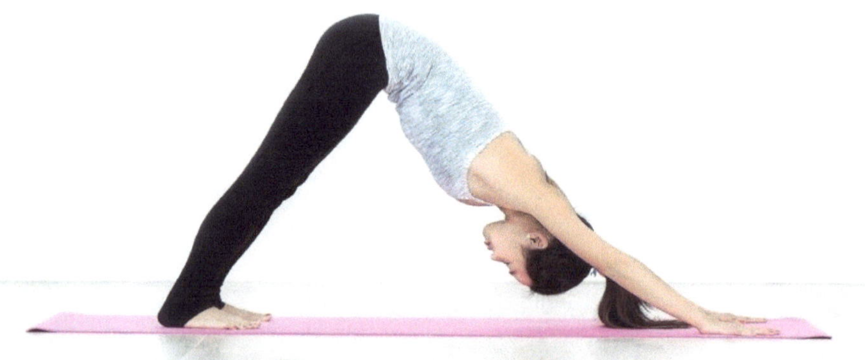

- **Benefits of Downward Facing Dog Pose:**
  - ➢ Stimulates various body system
  - ➢ Encourages blood flow, gives you a glow.
  - ➢ Can open up your sinus or other nasal congestions.
  - ➢ Relieves neck and back pain
  - ➢ Provides incredible balance of mind and body
- **How to do it?**
  - ➢ Get on all of your fours with hands and knees shoulder-and-hips-width apart.
  - ➢ Then walk on your hands forward and spread your fingers wide for stability.
  - ➢ Curl your toes under and carefully press your hips upward. Your body will look like an inverted V
  - ➢ Feet should be hip-width apart.
  - ➢ Knees slightly bent.

Warrior I (Virabhadrasana I):

Warrior I is a standing yoga pose that builds focus, power, and stability. It is an essential pose as it builds stamina in yoga practices.

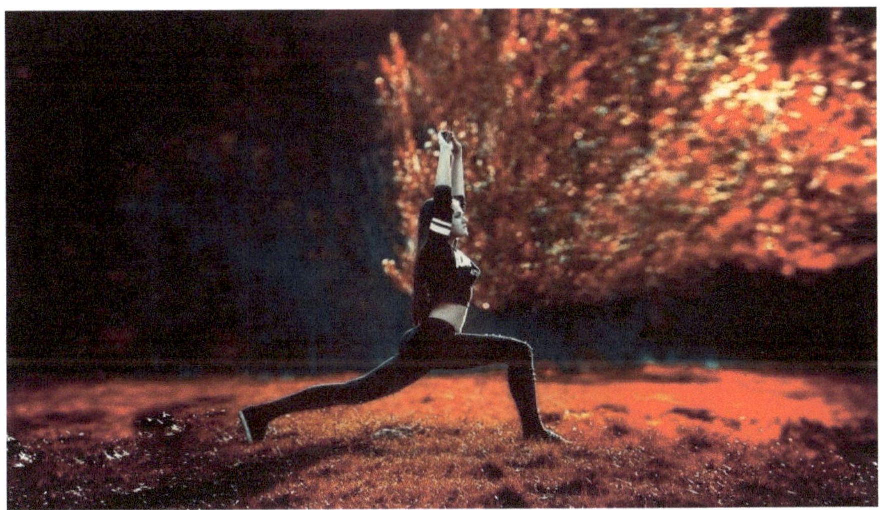

- **Benefits of Warrior I Pose:**
  - ➢ Strengthens your shoulders, arms, legs, ankles, and back
  - ➢ Opens your hips, chest, and lungs
  - ➢ Improves your balance
  - ➢ Encourages good circulation and respiration
  - ➢ Stretches your arms, legs, shoulders, neck, and belly
  - ➢ Uplifts and energizes the entire body
- **How to do it?**
  - ➢ From a standing position, step your left foot to the back of your mat.
  - ➢ Next, bend your right knee 90 degrees and straighten your back leg.
  - ➢ On your inhale, raise your arms above your head, so your palms are facing each other
  - ➢ Stay at least for 15 seconds
  - ➢ Slowly ease out your pose by lowering your arms and bring your legs back together.

Warrior II (Virabhadrasana II):

Compared to Warrior I, Warrior II offers minor variations with your upper body instead of facing forward, should be rotated to the side. This version of warrior pose is helpful in building up your stamina.

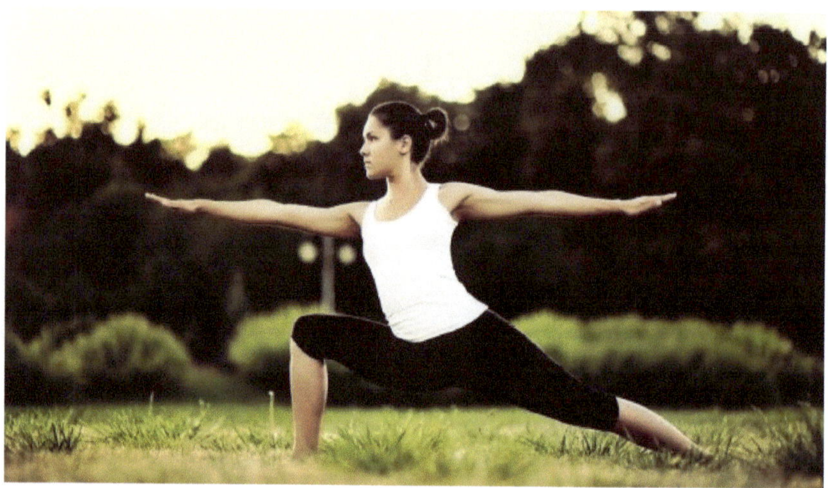

- **Benefits of Warrior II (Virabhadrasana II):**
  - ➤ Warrior II pose strengthens and stretches the legs and ankles.
  - ➤ It also helps to thoroughly stretch the chest, lungs, and shoulders.
  - ➤ Helpful in stimulating the abdominal organs and improves digestion.
  - ➤ Increase stamina
  - ➤ It releases any kind of backaches.
  - ➤ Promotes peace, courage, and auspiciousness.
- **How to do it?**
  - ➤ Stand completely straight and spread your legs about three to four feet apart.
  - ➤ Turn your right foot outwards by about 90 degrees and your left foot inwards by about 15 degrees.
  - ➤ Lift your arms sideways such that they are at your shoulder height. Make sure your palms are facing upwards.
  - ➤ Your arms should be placed parallel to the ground.
  - ➤ Take a deep breath, and as you exhale, bend your right knee.
  - ➤ Now, smoothly turn your head, and look to your right-hand side.
  - ➤ As you get comfortable in the pose, you need to push yourself further. Stretch your arms, and gently push your pelvis down.
  - ➤ Keep breathing.

> ➤ Inhale and come out of the pose. Drop your arms as you exhale.
> ➤ Repeat the pose on your left leg by turning your left foot outwards by 90 degrees and your right foot inwards by about 15 degrees.

Seated Twist (Ardha matsyendrasana):

Are you tired of sitting in the office for long running hours? Seated twist pose will offer you a great stretch that works perfectly for your shoulders, neck, and hips.

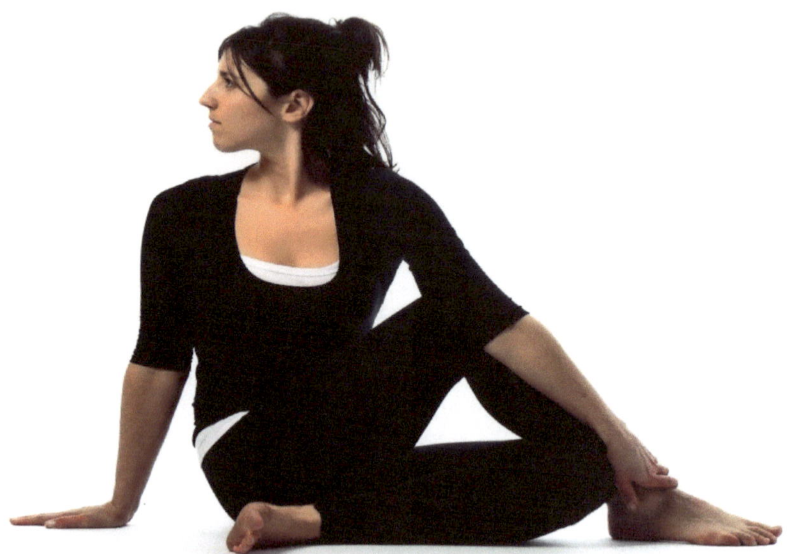

- **Benefits of Seated Twist:**
  - Provides flexibility to the spine
  - Burns fats from the abdomen
  - Beneficial in cases of slip disc
  - Effective in proper working of kidneys and liver
  - Useful in treating indigestion and constipation
  - Releases stress and strain
- **How to do it?**
  - Sit up with the legs stretched out straight in front of you.
  - Keeping the feet together and the spine erect.
  - Bend the left leg and place the heel of the left foot beside the right hip
  - Take the right leg over the left knee.
  - Place the left hand on the right knee and the right hand behind you.
  - Twist the waist, shoulders, and neck in this sequence to the right and look over the right shoulder.
  - Keep the spine erect.

➢ Hold and continue with long gentle breaths in and out.

Bridge Pose (Setu Bhanda):

Performing Bridge Pose makes you more alert in your mind. It is considered to be a great warm-up for more intense backbends

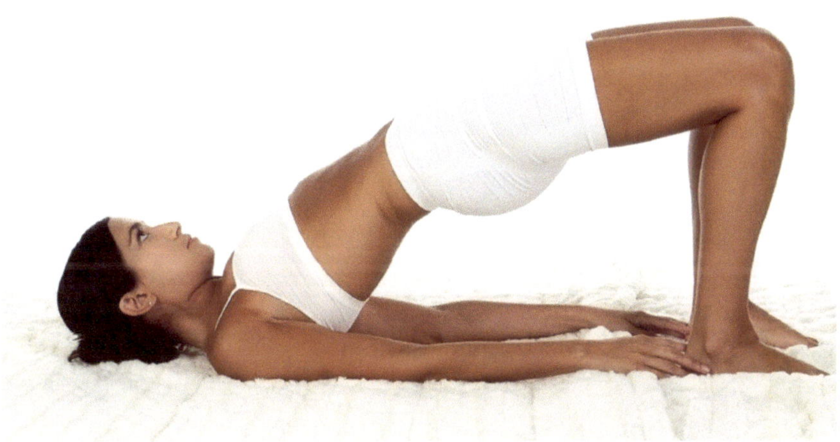

- **Benefits of Bridge Pose:**
➢ Improved Energy and Creativity
➢ Opens the heart chakra
➢ Relief During Menstruation
➢ Improves circulation of blood
➢ Helps alleviate stress and mild depression
➢ Calms the brain and central nervous system
➢ Reduces a backache and headache
➢ Eases fatigue, anxiety, and insomnia
- **How to do it?**
➢ Lay down on your back with your feet pressed into the floor and knees bent
➢ Extend your arms along the floor.
➢ Your palms should be flat.
➢ Exhale and lift your hips toward the ceiling.
➢ Roll your shoulders back and underneath your body.
➢ Hook your hands and extend your arms along the floor beneath your pelvis.
➢ Straighten your arms as much as possible.

- ➢ Keep your thighs and feet parallel.
- ➢ Hold for up to one minute.
- ➢ To release, untie your hands and place them palms-down alongside your body.
- ➢ Exhale as you slowly roll your spine along the floor.
- ➢ Allow your knees to drop together.

Corpse Pose (Shavasana):

Corpse Pose completely relaxes your body and mind. It is usually practiced at the end of a long active session of yoga.

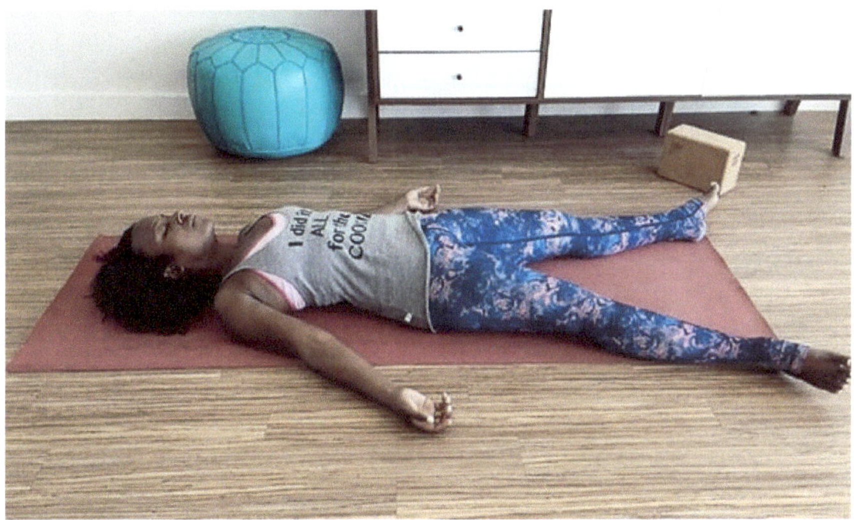

- **Benefits of Corpse Pose:**
  - ➢ Brings the body to a meditative state
  - ➢ Helps repair the cells and tissues and releases stress.
  - ➢ Reduces blood pressure and anxiety
  - ➢ Improves concentration and memory
  - ➢ Increases levels of energy
  - ➢ Boost energy and increases your productivity
- **How to do it?**
  - ➢ Lie flat on the floor.
  - ➢ Make sure there will be no disturbance for the duration of the pose.
  - ➢ Make yourself comfortable.
  - ➢ It is advisable to lie on a hard flat surface. Don't use any pillows or cushions.
  - ➢ Simply close your eyes.
  - ➢ Place your legs comfortably apart.
  - ➢ Your arms must be placed along your body and slightly apart
  - ➢ Your palms should be open and facing upwards.
  - ➢ Now, slowly pay attention to every area of your body, starting from your toes.

- ➢ As you do this, breathe slowly, yet deeply, setting your body in a state of deep relaxation.
- ➢ Keep all your focus on yourself and your body, forgetting all other tasks.
- ➢ Make sure you don't sleep
- ➢ After 10 to 15 minutes, roll to one side, keeping your eyes closed.
- ➢ Stay in the position for a minute, until you sit up again.
- ➢ Take a few deep breaths and gain awareness of your surroundings before you open your eyes.

Well, flexible body, relaxed mind, glowing skin, good health; whatever you are looking for, practicing Yoga is the best choice in every aspect. Yoga is truly an all-rounder that let you lead much calmer, happier and fulfilling life.

Section 2 – Introduction to Mindfulness

What is Mindfulness?

Mindfulness refers to the human ability to be fully present and maintain moment-to-moment awareness of the feelings, thoughts, body sensations and the surrounding environments deprive of any judgments – good or bad. It is a great way to introduce a little calmness into your life. Even small, simple techniques can bring about a tremendous change in your moods, and you are capable of better controlling your sentiments and actions.

What 'Mindfulness' basically involves is;

- Living in the moment
- Paying attention to what you think or feel without being judgmental
- Being fully alert of where you are and what you are doing
- Acceptance

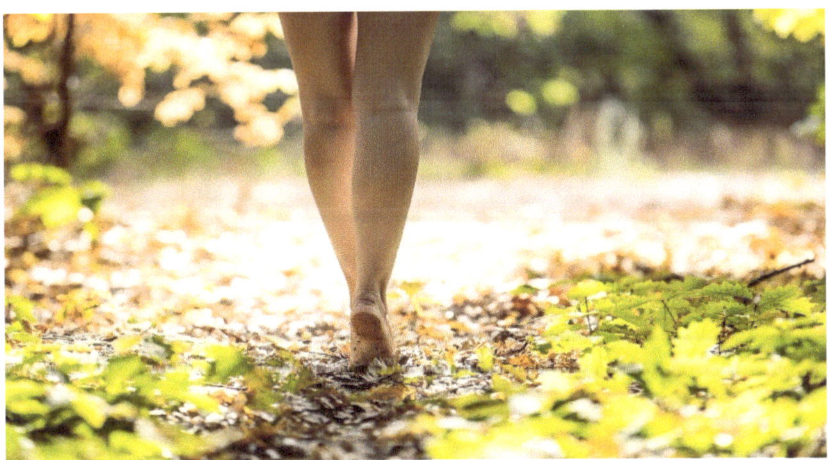

Human mind comprises emotional energies which tend to be powerful forces to fuel up our thoughts and beliefs. Gathering up and utilizing these strengths in a well responsive positive way is what that is entirely under our control. The way you perceive, interpret and react is all about the game of your mind, and YOU are the master of your own mind. Thus lingering on to your past or sitting anticipating your future will end up piling anxiety and worries for you which will lead you to become the slaves of your fears and emotions.

What are the core benefits of Mindfulness?

Incorporating Mindfulness into your daily routine life will definitely enhance and strengthen the range of astounding benefits that you are going to cultivate. Let us have a look at the calming and joyful experiences you will have by practicing Mindfulness and how it will bring about changes to your life.

- Decreases anxiety and stress levels as it shrinks the stress region in your brain.
- Lowers down the blood pressure and heart rate
- Increased immune system
- Reduces chronic pain
- Improve sleep
- Higher brain functioning
- Enhances the ability to deal with illness in a far better manner
- Ease gastrointestinal difficulties
- Improves eating disorders.
- Develops your working memory, concentration, and performance.
- Promotes self-awareness and overall well-being.
- Allows you to make better utilization of your strengths
- Encourages you to strongly deal with the hardships.
- Experience of feeling connected
- Better attention and focus
- Increased clarity in thinking and perception
- Adds up to the feeling of contentment and life satisfaction.
- Less emotional reactivity
- Relationship satisfaction
- Better quality of life

How can we practice Mindfulness?

Mindfulness practices do not require plenty of your time, although some patience and persistency is all that you need. Numerous ways are adopted to exercise Mindfulness. The goal is to achieve a focused relaxation by paying attention to your emotional state, considerations, and observations without criticism. This permits you to refocus and breathe in present moments. Let's explore the mindfulness techniques.

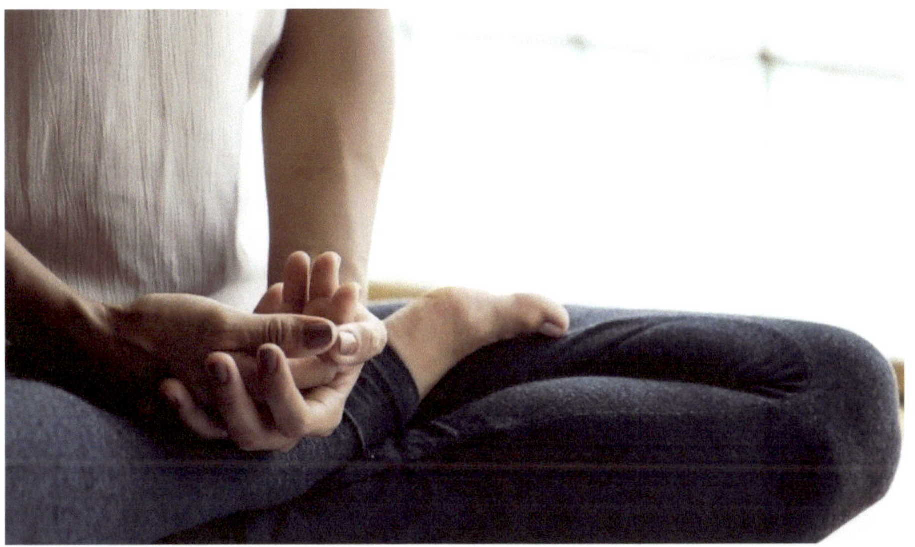

- Take a silent spot.
- Sit quietly on a comfortable, stable and solid chair, or you can sit cross-legs on the floor and focus on your natural breathing. Let the thoughts come and go but don't judge them. You may start reciting a mantra that you repeat silently.
- As you breathe, follow the vibes as the air goes in and comes out
- Feel your body sensations from head to toe successively and let them pass.
- A human mind is often carried away in thoughts. Be kind and gentle to yourself if you start to wander. Take a few minutes and then return your attention to breathing.
- Accept the presence of emotions and swiftly pass them away.

From sunrise till dawn, adding love and attention to every simple task of your daily routine, let you feel and enjoy the pleasures of every moment of your life. Have a look to some of it.

- While you walk around, 'walk mindfully.' Pay attention to every step you take. Walk as if you are kissing the ground and occasionally focus on the movement of your body and surroundings.
- Connect with your senses – sight, smell, taste, sound, and touch. For instance, pause and listen to the birds chirping in the morning, feel

the warmth of the coffee cup you hold; you will be amazed how much joy it will bring.
- When you eat, focus on what is in front of you. Relish the smell and taste of every bite of the scrumptious delight.

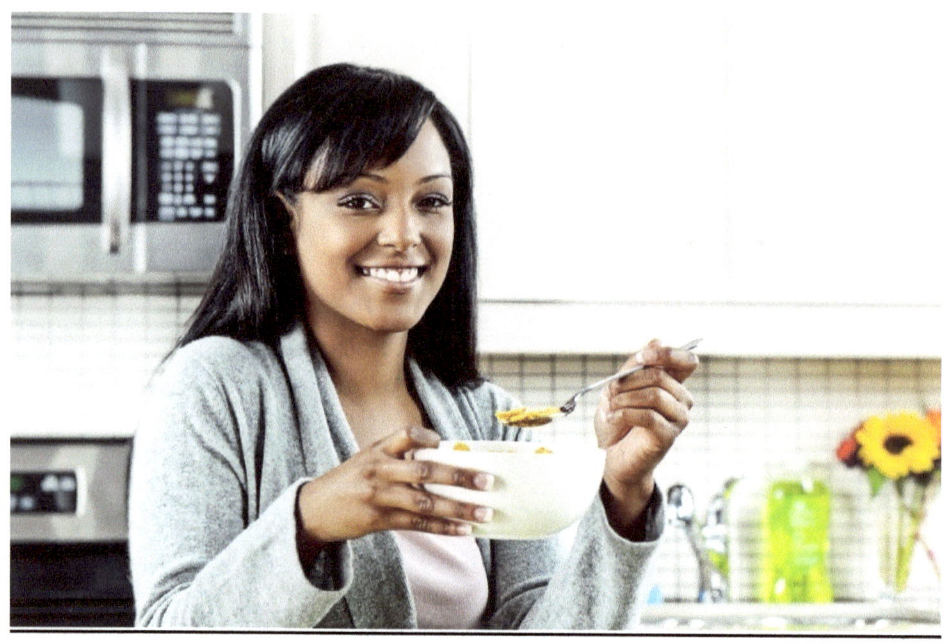

MINDFULNESS FOR WOMEN AND PREGNANCY

Becoming a mother is one of the most precious feelings that a woman ever feels. Undoubtedly, with every passing moment, the minds of mums-to-be are filled with endless queries and curiosities at the same time. Will my baby be healthy? Will I be able to take care of my child like good moms? How will the labor go? Will it hurt? And much more!!

Pregnancy can be overwhelming with body enduring so many changes as well as making decisions regarding birth plans, shopping stuff and a lot more. Practicing mindfulness can be a great way to keep your head high with a positive attitude and open mind to get through the challenges of pregnancy. Here are a few reasons why we suggest pregnant women to give it a try!

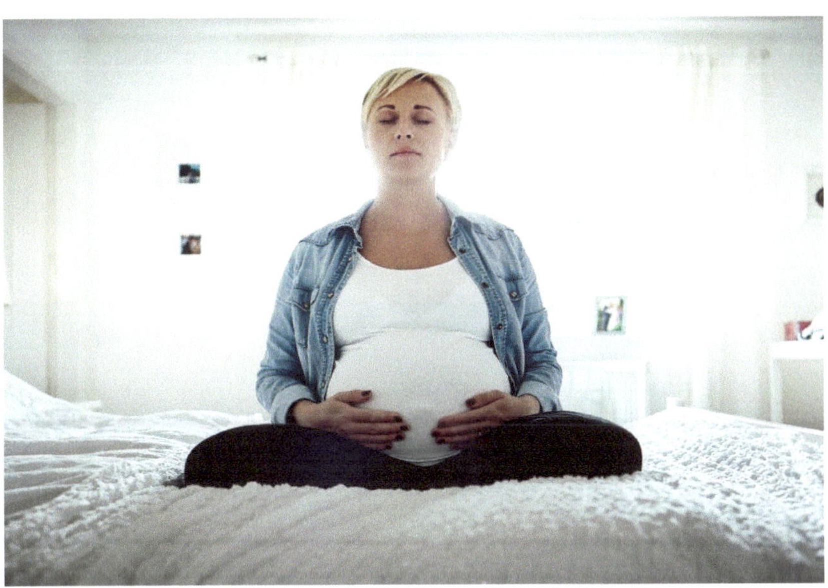

Reasons to practice mindfulness during pregnancy:

Helps you manage stress:

During pregnancy, women may undergo a lot of depression phases and serious anxiety attacks. A pregnant woman has to deal with a lot of discomforts which lead them to stressful situations. For better controls, researchers have suggested that Mindfulness can really help. Being in the moment can help pregnant women lower down their stress levels and keep their spirits high.

Ignites positive feelings:

Some pregnant women might expect pregnancy to be painful and exhausting. In doing so, they often overlook the warm and blissful moments. By being mindful, just notice your various body sensations during the whole day. Seriously you will simply love it, and it will lead you to boosted positive energies.

Helps you get a deep sleep:

It is difficult to get a good night sleep when you are pregnant. Taking time out for a Mindful session will let you have a fulfilling and deeper sleep.

Helps you to set up a healthy environment:

Well, of course, creating a healthy environment around the house for yourself and the baby to come is very beneficial. A quick mindful sitting will surely help you in this regard. Do not neglect your feeling and remember to express yourself openly.

Reduces pain during pregnancy and labor:

Doing 'Mindful Yoga' has proved to lessen the pains and twinges in case of a pregnant woman. Moreover, implementing such sort of activity at the time of labor pains also helps in coping with the pains effectively.

Strengthen the bonding with baby:

Mindfulness allows you to fully immerse yourself in quiet, soothing moments. What if it is you and your baby together? Feel every bit of a second and it will leave you with a sense of satisfaction, love, and completion; intensifying the attachment between you two. The strong bond with your baby is supportive during pregnancy and after as well. It helps you do well physically and emotionally with your child.

Helps to create strong relationships:

Women do get sensitive to petty issues when they are pregnant. Mindfulness helps in comforting their emotional state of mind. Take time out to consider others as well and be grateful for their help. Recognizing such people around you will help you win lifetime loving relationships.

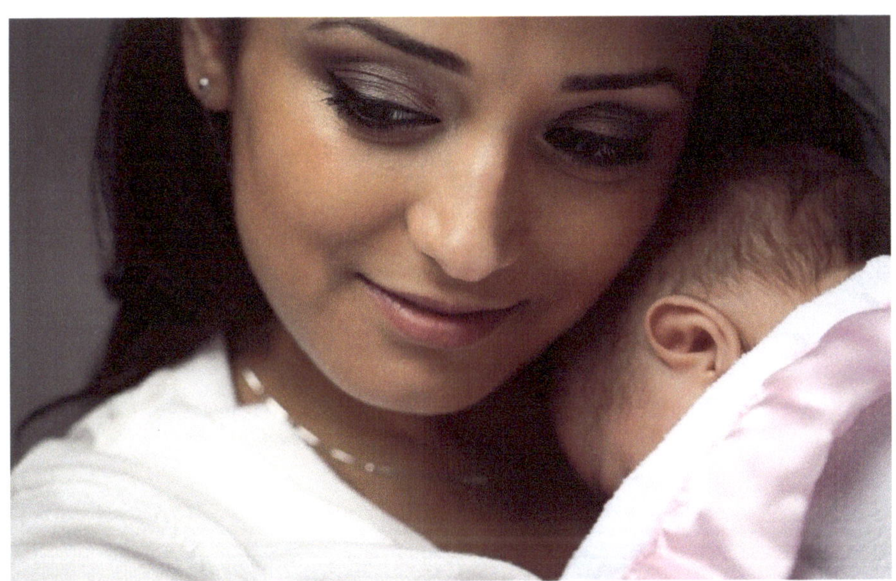

MINDFUL PARENTING
What is Mindful Parenting?

Mindful Parenting simply means to strive to make the best out of each moment you spend with your child. The ultimate goal is to remain 100% focused on them rather than thinking about what's going to be cooked tonight.

Time is running, and so are we. Stressed and overloaded with a lot of serious stuff, how can WE – as parents, can create a healthy environment for our kids at home if we are not fresh and peaceful in our minds, isn't it? Well, being a parent; probably the most precious gift that we can give to the children is our full presence. But before that, what I believe, we should be well aware of our own deepest needs. Nurture self-compassion and self-acceptance for ourselves.

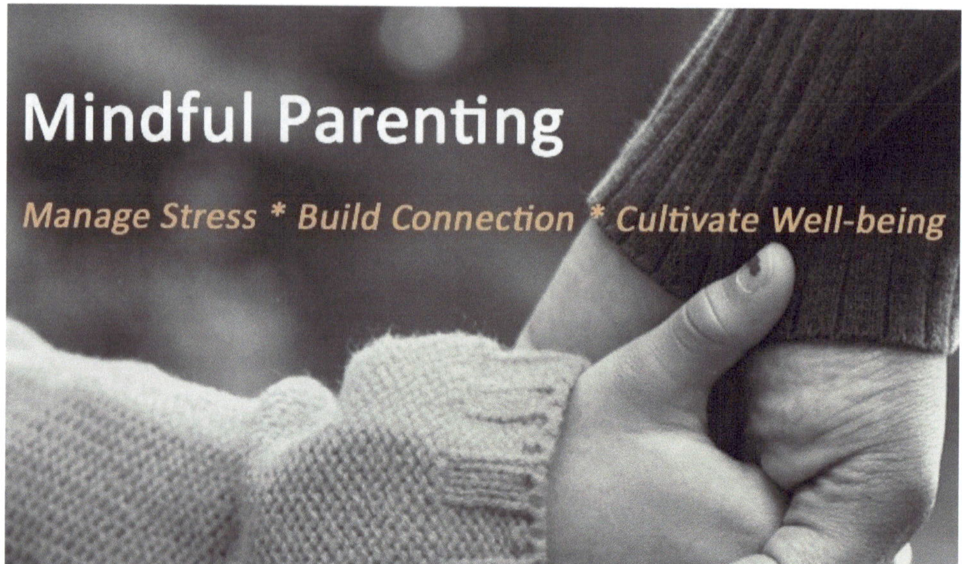

How can we rehearse to accomplish Mindful Parenting?

Make space for mindfulness in your lives. Experience the happening of every moment with a kind heart and vigorous acceptance. Only after this, we would be able to achieve effective mindful parenting.

- Find a quiet, dedicated place inside your house and reserve it for meditation and nothing else.
- Meditating together with your kids is one of the best possible practices.
- Avoid preoccupying your mind with the ideas that how your child is going to react to a certain situation. Take a step back. Appreciate each moment as it comes to you.
- As things do get chaotic in a house full of kids, do not over exert yourself. Take a few Mindful breaks.
- See the world through your child's eye. For instance, if your child comes running to you with a butterfly in hand, match his or her excitement and joy with yours.
- Routines are no doubt good for your children and are one of the key components to teach your child how to spend a well-organized life. But on the other hand, breaking these routines once in a while is perfectly fine. The time so spent mindfully with your child creates memories to cherish for a lifetime.

- Participate in the activity of their choice.
- Focus on self-care. We sometimes hesitate to enjoy the things that we use to do before we were parents. Stop doing that!! Indulge yourself in the activities you loved doing once. A healthier happier YOU will make you a healthier happier parent.

So, during our hectic routine life, the trick of mindfulness can calm us down and allow us to handle time to time hard situations easily. Well, I am talking about brief periods of time where we can focus on to what we hear, smell, taste, feel and even breathe. As we start paying attention even when we are frustrated or bored, eventually it becomes our habit which offers great help for staying focused even when our kids are nagging around.

Key advantages of Mindful Parenting:

- A deeper understanding of your own stressful responses
- Enriched ability to respond more skillfully to the unplanned and traumatic moments with your child
- Helps you to learn to listen to your child with kindness.
- Helpful in solving problems of your child with patience.
- Reduces your reactivity as we are dealing with the calm place of the mind
- Allows us to make better choices by accepting our child's needs.
- Promotes greater satisfaction attached to our parenting skills
- Stimulates strong, trusting relationship.
- Increases your child's emotional strength and well-being
- Improves your child's capacity to reply with gentleness to others
- Encourages healthier and more productive relationships with all the family members

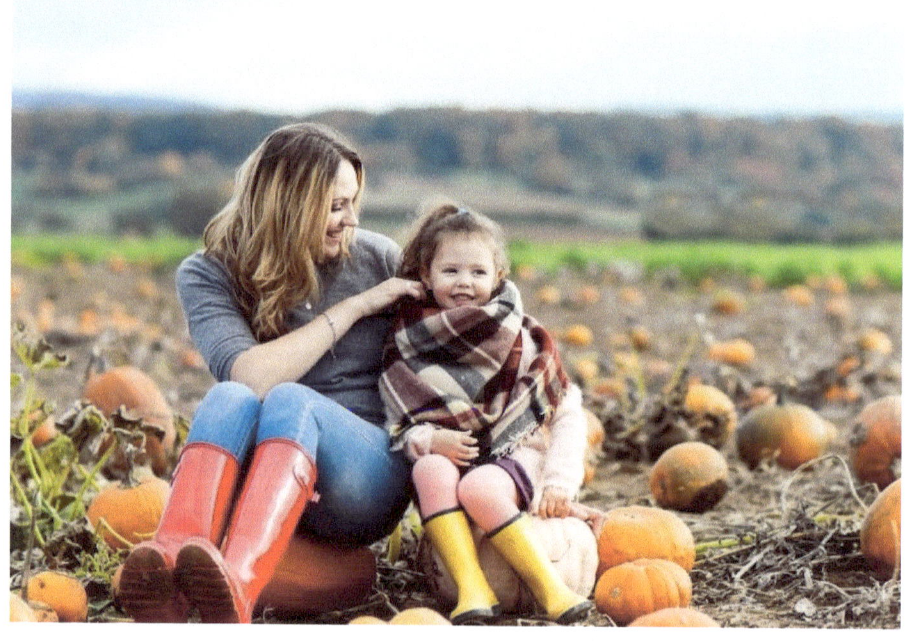

MINDFULNESS FOR CHILDREN

Coping and dealing with competitive environments of the present times, our children are forced to work pretty hard these days. They have somewhat become robotics in the quest of attaining victory. However, what I believe these innocent angels do not deserve to remain under pressures and lead a stressful life, at least at this point in their life.

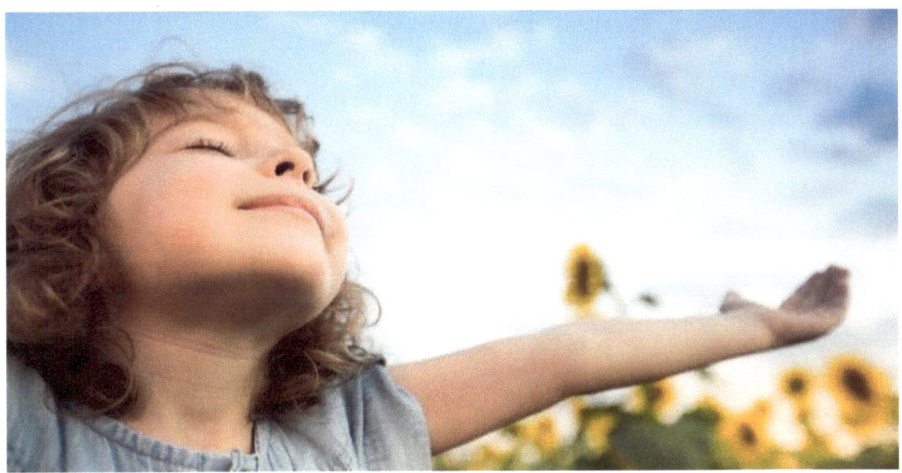

So, here we have compiled some mindfulness techniques for your children to teach them how to slow down for a while and observe what is happening in the present moments. Encourage them to stop and breathe; be in the moment and appreciate the blessings that surround them.

Mindful movements:

- Ask your children to walk around the room as stiff as a mummy. Funny! But a great activity to uncover how it really feels like moving with stiff arms and legs
- Next, tell your children to pretend like a falling leaf and glide through the air. Dig deep into the feel of this movement too.

Well, actually this sort of activity will help your children experience the difference between being tense and relaxed. Do not forget to put on some funky music in the background to add more joy to this entertaining activity.

Smell Me! What am I?

Take out all the herbs and spices from your kitchen cabinet and let your children smell them one by one. Ask them

- To guess what they are?
- Out of all the scents, which smell they remembered and liked the most?
- What that particular smell they liked, remind them of?

Have your children speak out and explain about different scents they smell.

Creating Sensory Bin:

- Take your children for a nature walk and ask them to collect different items related to nature.
- Now once you return, take a box marked as "Sensory Bin" and fill it with wonders of nature.
- Next, blindfold your children and ask them to take out an item from the bin.
- Feel it, smell it and guess what it is?

Playing guessing game with the nature items they are holding in their hands let them focus and to stay in present times.

Quick Mindful Exercises:

- Let your child blow bubbles. Focus on the bubble as they are blown, float and burst.
- Get your child a balloon to play. The balloon is then aimed to be kept off the ground.
- Ask your child to do fun posing that can make him feel focused, strong and happy.
- To develop focus and body awareness, request the child to focus his gaze at a point and stand on one leg. By adding Mindful Breathing, the balancing becomes easier.
- Take your child to the park and instruct to listen and count the sounds they hear silently like children playing around, sounds of moving swings, footsteps on dried leaves, birds singing, a man saying hello and much more.

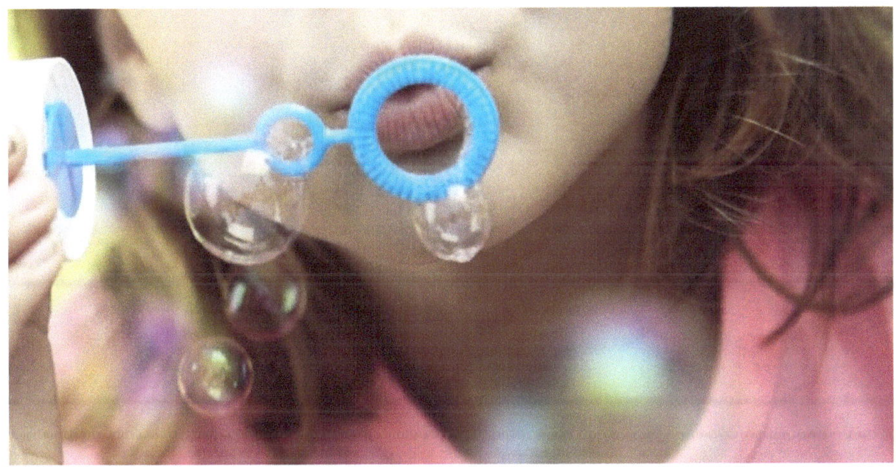

MEDITATION

What is meditation?

Nowadays, meditation is the most buzzed word. It isn't about becoming an entirely a different person or something; it is all about training yourself to attain a state of consciousness and giving a break to your mind. Well, this doesn't mean that you have to turn off your feelings and thoughts, but you need to observe them with clearer mind without judging anything.

Whatever you do with complete awareness is meditation which let you have a healthier perspective on the things happening in your life that will eventually lead you to have a better understanding of them. We all seek for happiness and deeper mental contentment, right? So, meditation is the perfect idea to cultivate pleasures and avoid sufferings.

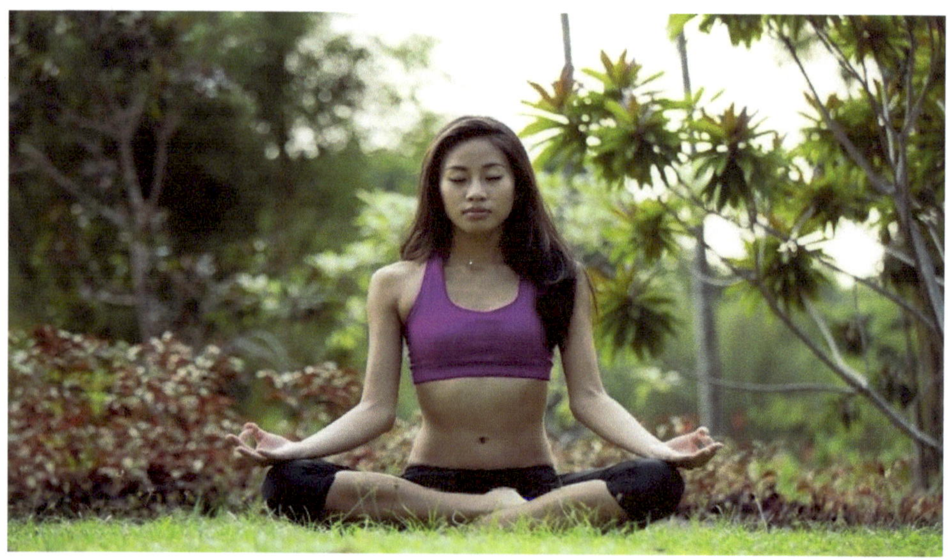

Why is meditation important?

Meditation is essential to feel fit and live a healthy life. It helps us in eliminating all the negative thoughts, worries, and anxieties that prevent us from being satisfied and happy. Making meditation part of our everyday life will make us feel fresh and handle difficult situations in a far better way. Here we list down the Psychological as well as the physical benefits of meditation.

Psychological benefits of meditation	Physical benefits of meditation
Soothes and comfort your mind	Stimulates your nervous system
Take away your worries	Slows your respiration for longer, deeper breaths.
Helps your control your anger	Decrease physical tensions
Boost your energy levels	Lowers your blood pressure
It makes you more tolerant	Strengthens your immune system
Brings clarity to your mind	Delete psychosomatic disorders caused by stress
Improves your confidence	Recharge your batteries
Encourages personal growth	Improves athletic performance
Calmness	Slows down the aging process

Tips to start a fruitful meditation:

- Try to meditate every day and possibly at the same time that may help you to become regular in meditating yourself.
- Avoid taking coffee before you meditate.
- Do not meditate immediately after meals. The best time to meditate is when you are not full of energy.
- Prepare a calm and quiet place where you will enjoy your meditation. You can open up a window for some fresh air flow.
- Choose a place not very bright.
- Wear comfortable clothes.
- It is very important that you are not disturbed during your meditation so close the door; disconnect your phone as it is a time of the day dedicated to yourself only.

If you want to feel good about yourself, start your meditation right away. Seriously, within a few minutes, you will feel a sense of self-control, freshness, and serenity penetrating deep down into your mind and heart. No doubt the beginners do find it difficult at the start but with the passage of time you are surely going to start loving it.

<u>**Summary**</u>

Thank you for reading I hope you have found some new exercises to try, which can help you relieve some stress. May you continue to live in a mindful way and be present in the moment, so that you can enjoy the simple pleasures of what life brings.

If you enjoyed this book please leave feedback, it would be very much appreciated.

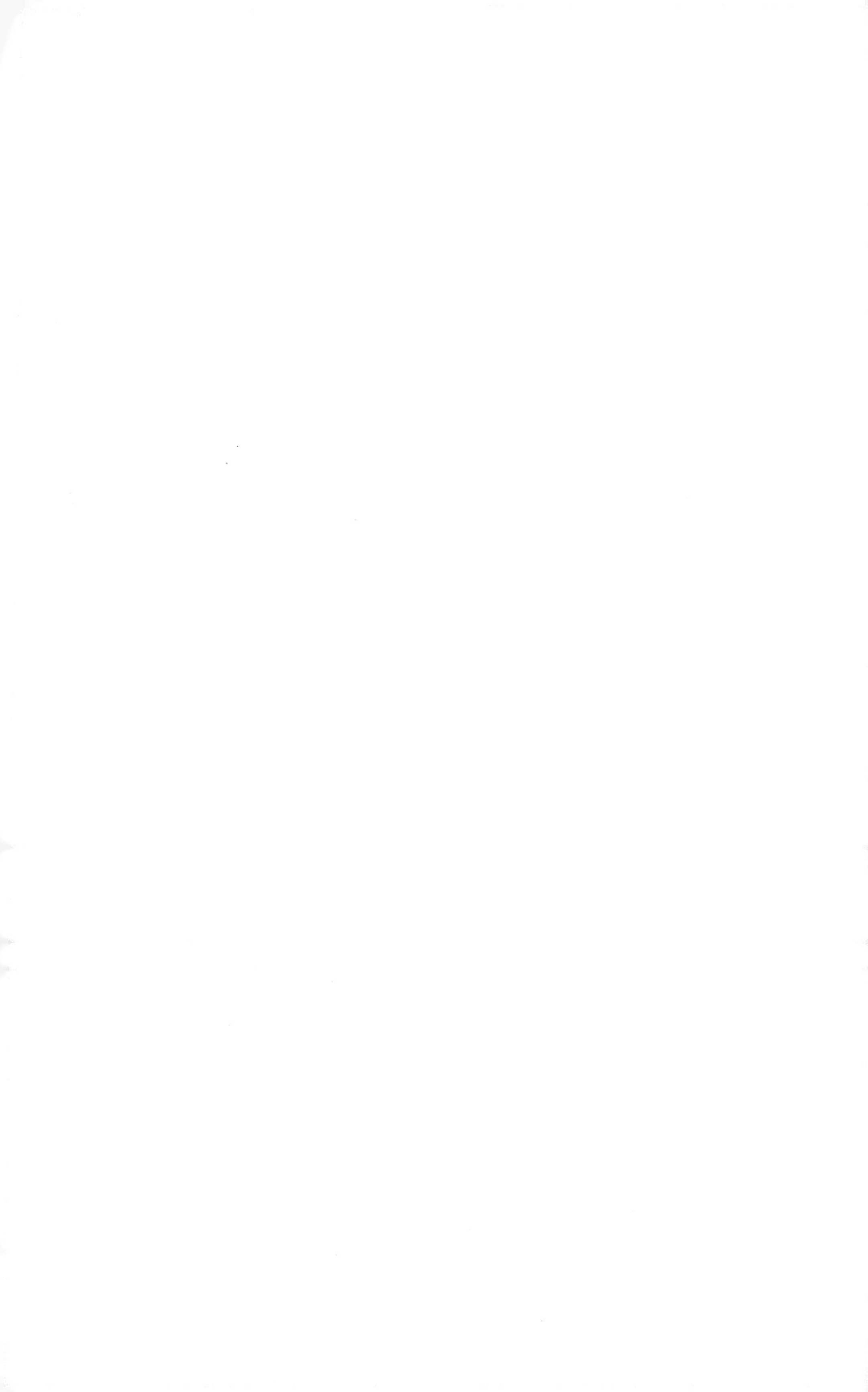